I0428484

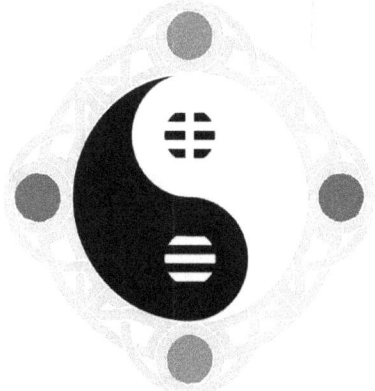

Seated Chi Baton Exercises

TM©

By Barry Westley

Published by Barnaby Jay Publications

Copyright © Barry Westley 2014

Barry Westley asserts the moral right to be identified as the author of this work.

All rights reserved. No part of this publication may be reproduced, stored in a retrieval system, or transmitted in any form, or by means, electronic, mechanical, photocopying, recording or otherwise, without the prior permission of the publishers.

Photographs by Kevin Laidler.

Cover designs by Graham Hodgson and Barry Westley.

This book is dedicated to:

Bob Szpalek (1951-2008). A man of huge physical, mental and spiritual gifts. I am forever grateful for his friendship, and miss him.

Also, with special thanks to:

My wife, Louise (for her endless, loving support).

Graham Hodgson, (the rock on whom I lean, for all my technical help).

&

Kevin Laidler for his patience and photographic skill.

Contents

Important Information

Chi Baton™ *exercises are very safe, but you should always consult your doctor before beginning any new exercise regime! If you have any doubts about the suitability of any of the exercises, you* **must** *refer back to your doctor, or medical practitioner, before attempting them!*

Do not do these exercises if you have been advised against them by your medical practitioner!

Follow the instructions carefully and do not rush, or "bounce", when performing any movement, or part of any movement!

Do the exercises at a pace that is comfortable for you and only do the number of repetitions that you can **easily** *handle. Build up slowly. You should feel refreshed after each of the programmes, not sore and exhausted! Be patient and you will progress more quickly!*

If you feel pain, when performing one of the movements, stop exercising and consult your doctor immediately!

It is also wise to wait at least six weeks before starting, or re-commencing, exercise after giving birth.

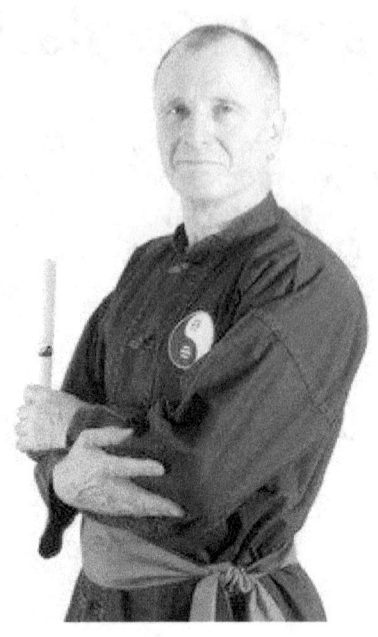

Introduction

Welcome to *Chi Baton*™ exercises.

Chi Baton™ exercises, (formerly known as *Chi-Baton Yoga* ™, and *Tai Rod Exercise System*™) is a series of special exercises which are performed using a short baton and are unique to me, **Barry Westley***.

Drawing on my extensive knowledge of **Taoist Yoga**, **Tai Chi Ch'uan, Powerlifting**, and a number of different martial arts, (both "hard" and "soft"), I have fashioned an extensive programme of low-impact, rhythmic exercises that strengthen the physical and energetic structure of the body.

Originally devised as a way of teaching principles of body mechanics in a simplified way to my students, *Chi Baton*™ proved to be popular, great fun and surprisingly effective in building internal energy, strength, stamina and flexibility.

Although, *Chi Baton*™ programmes were originally intended for myself and my immediate students, interest in this simple but effective system has grown to such an extent that I felt compelled to commit the exercises to record. Each programme can be used on its own or as a compliment to other *Chi Baton*™ programmes.

The *Seated Chi Baton*™ *Programme,* arose out of my work with **Age Concern/AgeUK**, and the need to develop a programme of exercises for those who had less flexibility, or were confined to a chair.

However, because the hips are anchored when sitting, many of my fitter, able bodied students love the *Seated Chi Baton*™ *Programme,* too. It does not allow them to cheat when performing the movements and can deliver a surprisingly effective workout even where space is strictly limited. Although devised as a workout for students with specific needs, *Seated Chi-Baton*™, has turned out to be a programme suitable for all.

The Baton

A *Chi Baton*™ is a piece of wood twelve and a half inches long which is held between the palms during exercise. (The length is of crucial importance as it gives the correct angles when exercising.)

It may also be made of copper or a mixture of copper and wood, or plastic and copper.

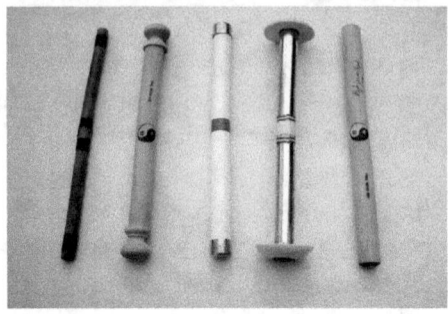

The easiest way to construct a **Chi Baton** ™ is simply to cut a piece of doweling the correct length (12 and a half inches, or 318 millimetres, and sand the cut ends.)

A _Chi Baton_™ is not to be confused with a Tai Chi Ruler which is a different length and, to my knowledge, used in quite a different way.

A simple **Chi Baton**™ is illustrated above. (I like to tap upholstery tacks in each end to contact the

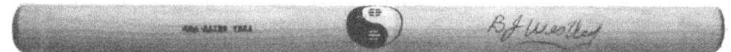

acupuncture points in the palm, but the baton works perfect well without them.)

Although this **Chi Baton** ™ is perfectly adequate, some students prefer to make their own of varying degrees of complexity.

However, the important principle is that the baton is comfortable, the correct length, and that you continue to use the same rod each time you exercise. In this way it becomes part of you and infused with your energy, increasing the power of your practice.

(***Barry Westley** has studied **Li Style Tai Chi Chu'an** and **Taoist Yoga** for over 26 years and is a black jacket instructor **(3rd Tengchi)**

He is also a black jacket instructor in **Feng Shou Kung Fu (1st Tengchi),** is a qualified referee in **Tui Shou ("Pushing Hands.")** and **Chinese Martial Forms**, has competed in National Tui Shou Competitions and has represented **England** in the sport of **Powerlifting**.

Barry Westley is also an ex **Shiatsu Practitioner** and ex **Associate Member of Malvern College of Healing**.)

Basic Principles of Chi Baton™ Exercises

N.B. When learning the exercises do not overload yourself trying to remember all of the principles below at one time. Learn the exercises thoroughly and gradually introduce each improvement when you feel it is appropriate to you. You will still derive considerable benefit from the exercises even if you forget some of the principles, provided you do not compromise the safe execution of the movements. Always remember, your energy will flow much better when you are relaxed. It is particularly important that you don't let technical considerations spoil your enjoyment of the programmes.

The principles of **Chi Baton™** are similar to those of Tai Chi Ch'uan and Taoist Yoga, **with some significant variations.** Although detailed instruction will be given for each exercise, it is wise to keep in mind the following:

1. **Head is held erect** as if being lifted slightly through the crown.

(This can be practiced by placing the tip of the nose against the wall and lengthening the back of the neck without allowing the nose to move.)

When seated, endeavor to keep the body upright, with a straight spine.

2. **Shoulders are relaxed**.

Even when raising arms above the head the shoulders stay down, using the ball and socket joint of the shoulders to effect the movement rather than lifting the shoulders upwards. The simplest way to achieve this effect is to imagine that your hand is resting on a balloon that is gradually inflating and rising up to lift the relaxed arm (i.e. "weight underside"). In this way, the correct muscles are used to lift the arm, and the elbows remain soft and without tension.

If both arms are raised at the same time, it is important to look up, allowing the chin to drift forward slightly as you do so, as this relieves the pressure on the blood vessels in the neck.

3. **Joints are never fully locked.**

Even where the arms and legs are straight, the elbows and knees are not fully locked. It should be possible to move easily from one movement to another without having to "release a joint."

4. **Tongue is placed on the roof of the mouth.**

Generally the tongue is placed on the roof of the mouth, just behind the front teeth, during the "expression" phase of a movement. The tongue is dropped from the mouth as the body "releases."

In this way, *Chi Baton*™ differs from many forms of Chinese Yoga and Tai Chi Ch'uan, where the tongue remains on the roof of the mouth at all times.

In *Chi Baton*™, the intention is that the energy pulses

as in an "alternating" current electric charge, rather than continuously flowing as in a "direct" current. (It is my personal belief that performing the exercises in this way makes them more dynamic and powerful).

The "expression" may take place in either the in or out breath of a movement, or in some cases, the expression and release may take place during a single breath.

5. **Weight is evenly spread over the whole area of the foot.**

Although there is less feeling of "weight" on the feet than when doing the standing exercises, the same principles should still apply. What weight there is should be evenly spread over the following areas; the heel, outside edge of the foot, both sides of the ball of the foot and the five toes.

(Obviously there will be less weight on the little toe than the heel, but all elements of the foot should feel as if they are equally contributing to the stability of the legs).

(In certain exercises the heel or toe is raised and then, of course, this principle will not apply.)

6. **During the majority of *Chi Baton*™ movements the waist turns independently of the hips.**

This ensures that the feet remain planted firmly and the knees remain in line with the feet. It also ensures that the correct strengthening movement is performed.

When performing the waist twists, the hips should remain facing forwards, so that abdomen rotates inside the bowl of the pelvis, rather like a globe revolves in its stand.

Although labelled a "waist twist", the movement is better described as a ***"central core body movement"***. This movement should originate deep within the bowl of the pelvis, and spiral upwards through the torso. The spine should remain straight and not twisted throughout. If the spine twists, the movement is not starting deep enough in the pelvis, the movement is too large, or the shoulder is drawing too far backwards and losing its connection with the turn of the waist.) .

7. The *Chi Baton*™ movements are performed in an even-paced rhythmic manner.

Although there is some flexibility in the actual speed of performing the movements, once that speed is decided upon it must be maintained throughout the programme.

That is, there should be no speeding up or slowing down, when performing an individual movement. In this way the maximum strengthening effect is safely produced with the minimum effort.

Ideally the ***Chi Baton***™ should be continually moving, without pauses. (For example, where a movement involves the arms extending outwards and then drawing inwards, it is best to put in a tiny loop at the extreme of each movement to ensure that the ***Chi Baton***™ continues to move at all times and that there is not a pause when the baton changes direction).

Generally, in my ***Chi Baton***™ classes, the movements are timed to a metronome set at 60 beats per minute.

Each movement usually taking four beats. If you do not possess a metronome, simply counting the beats "one and two and three…etc.") is perfectly adequate.

Programmes can also be performed at a livelier pace (roughly 72 beats per minute), for a more cardio vascular workout, or at a rhythmic pace to suit you. The important principle is that the exercises are not performed too quickly and that the movements do not speed up or slow down. It is important to resist this temptation as it will slow down progress.

8. **Perform the exercises in the order they are given.**

This is important, as many of the exercises act as a "warm   up" for the next exercise or as a counterbalance, or "cooling down" for a previous one. It is also important to complete the whole programme so do not exhaust yourself on the earlier ones so that you can not complete the full balanced programme.

9. **Express and Release during each exercise.**

The *expression* can come on either the **in**, or **out** breath, depending on the exercise.

During the *expression* phase one or more of the following should be present. (In an ideal world, of course, the student should introduce each element of the expression at the appropriate point of the exercise.):

a)   There is a gradual **slight** gripping of the toes, causing the instep to rise slightly, and stimulate the kidney 1 ("bubbling springs") acupuncture point in the

14

foot. The best way to perform this is to try to raise the instep slightly, and spread the bones of the feet sideways. In this way, the toes will grip naturally and not "over claw".

(Obviously, it is not appropriate to grip the toes if you are performing certain actions, such as raising your heels.)

In certain exercises, you may be required to express with only **one foot**, or **one hand**, or express different elements at different times. (This will be clearly indicated during the instructions for that exercise).

b) Gradually and <u>gently</u> contract the anal sphincter.

c) Stretch the central core of the body gently, gradually upwards to the crown of the head. (Before stretching upwards, focus on softly rolling the belly upwards and backwards, as this will allow the spinal stretch to be performed more easily.)

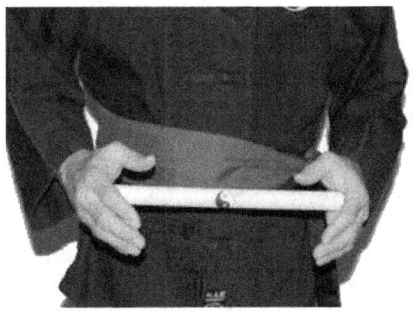

d) Normally the hands are relaxed as if holding a football, with the fingers gently touching each other, and the thumb at a forty-five degree angle.

*(When we talk of **relaxation**, in this manual, it is not the same as **collapse**. That is, when relaxed, the structure is still held and the tendons "engaged". It is*

deep relaxation without "floppiness". This is a difficult concept, and will take some practice to find the correct balance between tension and flaccidity.)

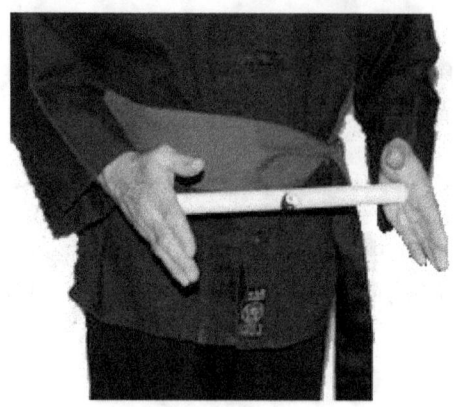

During the **expression** phase of a movement the fingers gently lengthen as if holding a slightly curved box. At the same time the thumb draws back until it is almost in line with the hand, and the bones of the hand are opened sideways. This should slightly increase the pressure at the end of the **Chi Baton**™ and activate the energy centre in the palm. (For this reason, **Chi Batons**™ of my design have a small stud in each end, to improve this contact.) Another way to achieve this expression in the hands is to imagine your hands are partly inflated balloons that further inflate, expand and lengthen during the **expression** phase.

e) The tongue gently contacts the roof of the mouth, just behind the teeth at the start of the **expression** phase.

During the **release** phase, everything gradually returns to the fully relaxed, start position, with the tongue no longer on the roof of the mouth. .

10. **Breathe in through the nose and out through the mouth.**

Breathe naturally in to the belly, the movement of the *Chi Baton*™ will direct the breath where it needs to be.

Remember that sometimes the exercise will make the breathing easier to perform (as for a Buddhist breath) and at other times the exercise will seem to make breathing more difficult (as for a Taoist compression breath). Both types of exercise are equally valid.

In some exercises both types of breathing are present.

11. **In general, keep weight "underside".**

When raising and lowering any part of the body while performing a movement of the *Chi Baton*™, direct your attention to the underside (that is, the side nearest the ground.)

This will produce a heavy sensation in the limb or body so that the action is both more relaxed and yet slightly more challenging. One way of understanding "weight underside" is to imagine that a balloon is inflating under the part of the body to be lifted. When lowering that part of the body imagine it is resting on a slowly deflating balloon.

Doing the exercises in this way has a more profound effect on the body's energy system and so you may feel tired for a while after exercising, until your body becomes accustomed to it.

*

N.B. Although it is not within the scope of this manual, it is a very good idea to "stretch out" after every workout programme.

Almost every movement in *Chi Baton*™ contains a large element of stretching, but spending a few extra minutes on held (but not forced), medium range, stretches will pay dividends, helping prevent excess lactic acid build up in the muscles.

The Chi Baton™ Logo

TM ©

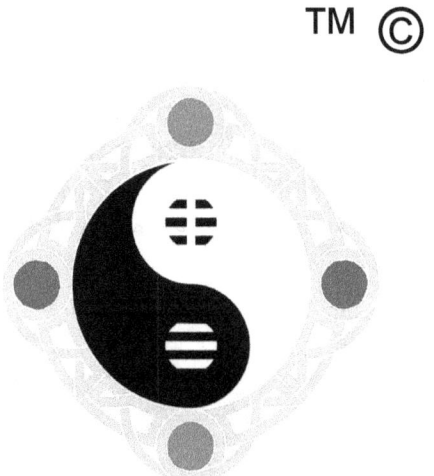

In developing the *Chi Baton*™ system of exercises I decided to design and adopt a specific Logo that reflected the spirit and aims of these exercises.

As the bulk of the exercises were based on the the Taoist system of Chinese Yoga and Chi Kung, I based the logo on the well known Yin and Yang symbol.

To further emphasise the spiritual aspect of this work, I cast the I Ching and came up with the hexagram T'ai.

This struck me as particularly relevant, not least because of the strong links *Chi Baton*™ has with T'ai Chi Ch'uan.

I decided to combine these to symbols to create, what I feel, is a logo of profound meaning and deep spiritual power.

19

In the logo, as in the I Ching, T'ai is for Peace, Harmony and Benevolence. With the trigram for earth (three black broken yin lines) being placed over the trigram for sky (three unbroken white yang lines). The sky intermingles with the earth. This is a very fortunate symbol. (Literally, "Heaven on Earth")

It is also about the strong supporting the weak, doing the right thing at the right time, and small offerings bringing large rewards. ("Less is more" to paraphrase the great Taoist book "The Tao Te Ching").It is about the strong and rigid force creating harmony with the weaker by being flexible and yielding.

My good friend, Chris Van Dyke, designed the knot work that surrounded it which represents the movement of the Tao, and is suffused with mathematical symbollism.

The exercises within this book were devised through intense study, together with meditation, dowsing and channeling, so a spiritual thread runs through them all. It is my personal belief that regular practice of these exercises can benefit an individual on the mental and spiritual levels as well as on the purely physical. I hope in time you will feel able to agree.

ChiBaton™ Programmes

This manual contains the basic **Seated Chi Baton**™ programme. This was developed mainly for those with limited ability, or fitness. (However, it does provide a complete workout for all.)

In the case of students who have a paralyzed limb, still attempt to move that limb. "Energy follows thought", and just thinking and making an effort will effect the overall balance of the body's energy, as well as exercising other companion muscle groups.

The same principle applies to those with a missing limb. Imagine moving that "ghost" limb to retain the bi-lateralism of the exercise.

(Although this programme is entire unto itself, if you enjoy it and want to learn more, you may be interested to know that there are other complete *Chi Baton*™ programmes planned for the future, should demand warrant. Details will be posted on the website: www.chibaton.co.uk)., or on Amazon's website.

Each exercise will contain a suggested number of repetitions, but obviously the student can perform more or less repetitions. The important thing is that you do not overtax yourself! (You should feel refreshed, not exhausted at the end of the session).

You should perform a roughly equal amount of repetitions for each exercise so that the programme retains its balance.

© ™

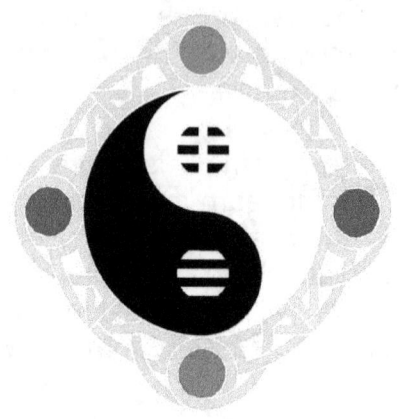

Seated Chi Baton™ © Programme

Seated Programme

Sit Still.

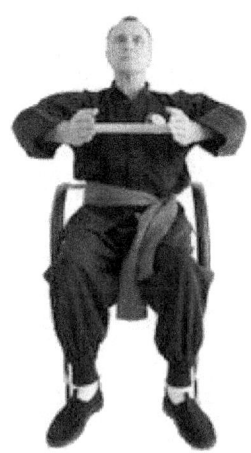

Sit comfortably, holding the rod at chest height, with the shoulders and elbows relaxed. Gently raise the elbows as if they have been lifted by balloons. As you lift the elbows, draw them outwards to ensure that the shoulder blades remain spread. Keep the tongue on the roof of the mouth and focus on circulating energy from the heart down the left arm, across the **Chi Baton** ™, up the right arm and through the body making a circle.

*(If you are inexperienced in visualizing energy, you may find it helpful to imagine warm water flowing down the arm and through the baton back to the heart. Persevere in visualizing until you can actually **feel** the movement of energy.)*

Do this for at least a minute to energise the heart and prepare the body for the work that follows.

Open the Fountain

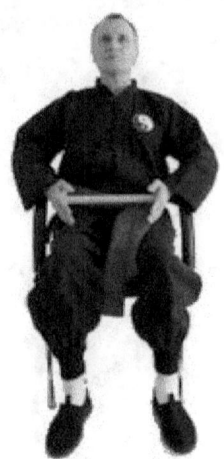

Sit comfortably, holding the baton, with the shoulders and elbows relaxed.

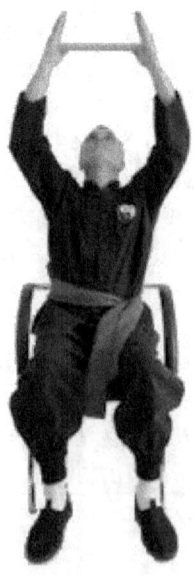

As you breathe in, *express* , as you lift the *Chi Baton*™ gently upwards, keeping it about one fist distance from the body, until it is above and slightly to the front of the head.

As you lift the **Chi Baton**™ gently upwards, draw the elbows outwards, allowing the shoulder blades to spread, so that the back is open. Follow the movement of the **Chi Baton**™ with your eyes as it travels past, and above, your face. Allow the chin to drift forwards a little as you do so, to ensure the blood vessels in the neck are kept free and open. Be careful not to compress the back of the neck, or arch your back, when performing this action.

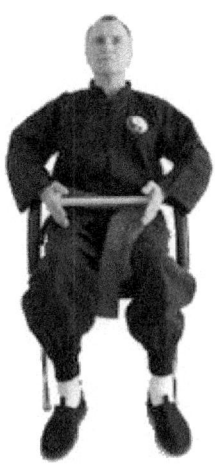

As you breathe out, *release*, in a controlled manner, and return to the start position, by rolling the shoulder joints so that the hands form a downward arc as they drop. At the same time relax the hands and feet, and allow the elbows to draw inwards and point downwards.

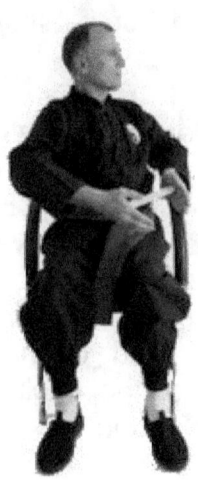

Without altering the position of your hips and buttocks, rotate your central core and turn your body, gently, to the left.

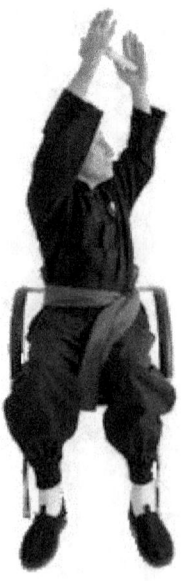

Keeping the body turned, breathe in and, **express** , as you lift the **Chi Baton**™ gently upwards, as before, keeping it about one fist distance from the body, until it is above and slightly to the front of the head.

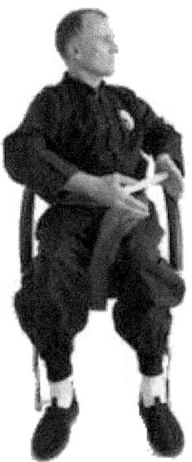

As you breathe out, **release**, in the controlled manner outlined in the previous movement.

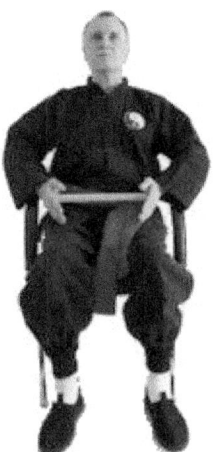

Return to the start position, facing forwards.

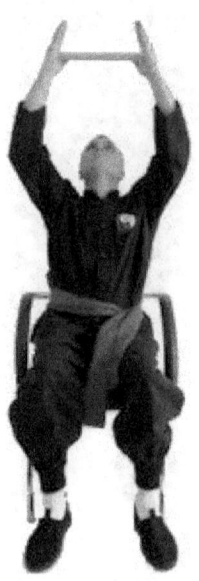

Breathing in, perform another repetition of the movement to the front.

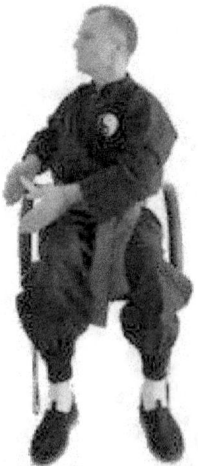

Without altering the position of your hips and buttocks, rotate your central core and turn your body, gently to the right.

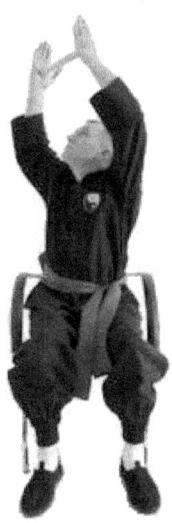

Perform another repetition of the movement to the right hand side, remembering to watch the movement of the *Chi Baton*™ as it travels past the face.

Turn back to the front position, and perform another repetition of the movement to the front.

Repeat the whole sequence outlined above another three times.

Raise Alternate Arms

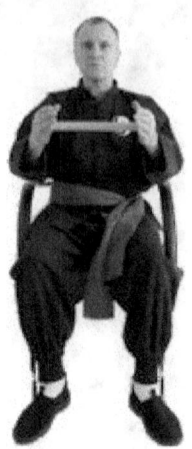

Sit comfortably, holding the baton at chest height, with the shoulders and elbows relaxed.

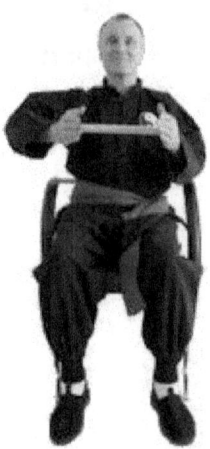

As you breathe in, **express** , as you lift the right elbow gently upwards, being careful to keep the shoulders down. The right forearm should almost form a straight line with the **Chi Baton**™

As you lift the elbow, draw it outwards to ensure that the shoulder blades remain spread.

(In this exercise, as you raise the right elbow, **express**
with the right hand and right instep only.)

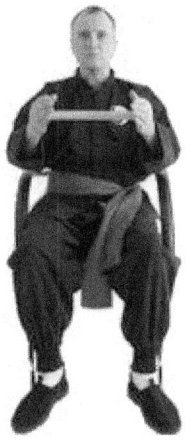

As you breathe out, **release**, in a controlled manner,
and return to the start position.

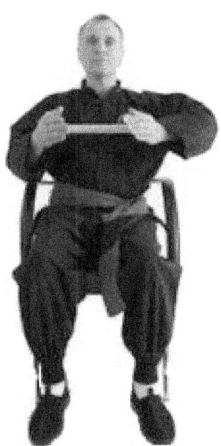

As you breathe in, repeat the expression, substituting
left for right.

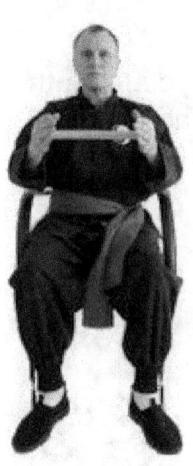

Return to the start position and repeat the whole sequence another three times.

Combined Alternate Arms

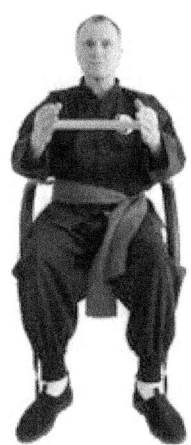

Sit comfortably, holding the rod at chest height, with the shoulders and elbows relaxed, but not floppy.

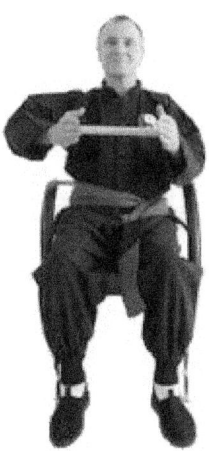

As you breathe in, with half your in breath, *express* , as you lift the right elbow gently upwards, being careful to keep the shoulders down. The right forearm should almost form a straight line with the **Chi Baton™**.

As you lift the elbow, draw it outwards to ensure that the shoulder blades remain spread.

(In this exercise, as you raise the right elbow, **express** with the right hand and right instep only.)

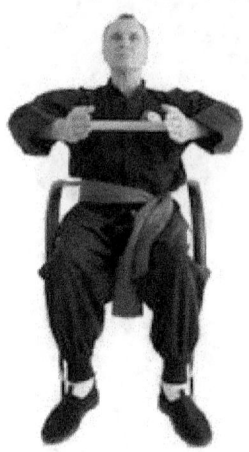

.
Continue to breathe in, as you **express**, and lift the left elbow gently upwards, so that both forearms form a straight line with the **Chi Baton™**. As you lift the elbow, draw it outwards to ensure that the shoulder blades remain spread.

(As you raise the left elbow, **express** with the left hand and left instep only.)

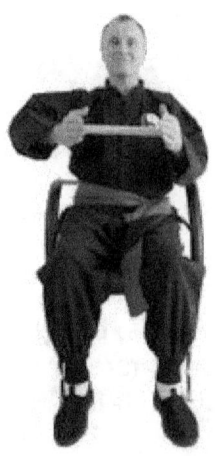 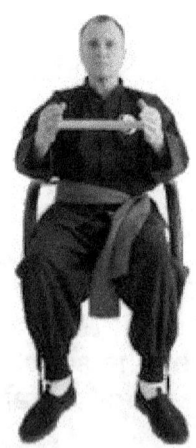

.
As you breathe out, **release**, in a controlled manner,

first lowering the left, then right elbows to return to the start position. (As you release each elbow, release the appropriate instep and hand.)

Repeat the whole of the above sequence.

Perform the exercise twice more, this time starting with the left.

Raise Both Arms

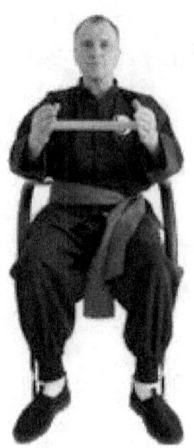

Sit comfortably, holding the rod at chest height, with the shoulders and elbows relaxed, but not floppy.

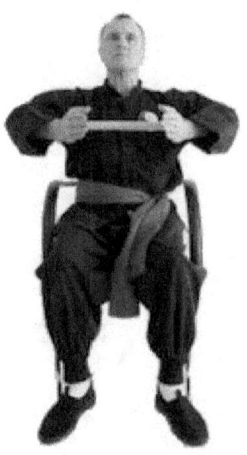

As you breathe in, **express** , as you lift both elbows gently upwards, being careful to keep the shoulders down. The forearms should almost form a straight line with the **Chi Baton™**. As you lift the elbows, draw them outwards to ensure that the shoulder blades remain spread.

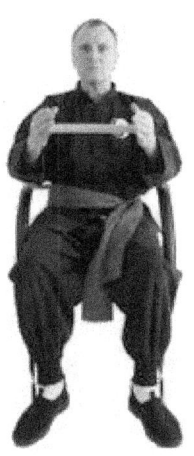

As you breathe out, **release**, in a controlled manner, and return to the start position.

Repeat the whole sequence another three times.

Drive The Hand Under

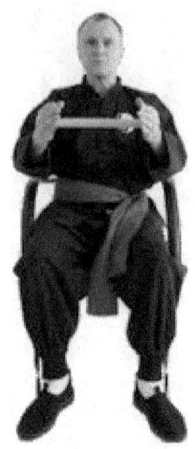

Sit comfortably, holding the rod at chest height, with the shoulders and elbows relaxed.

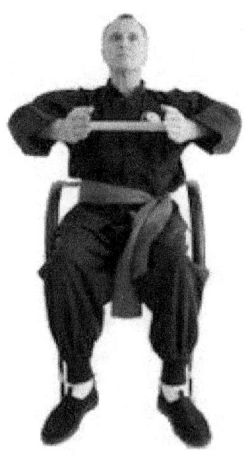

As you breathe in, lift both elbows gently upwards, being careful to keep the shoulders down. The forearms should almost form a straight line with the **Chi Baton™**. As you lift the elbows, draw them outwards to ensure that the shoulder blades remain spread.

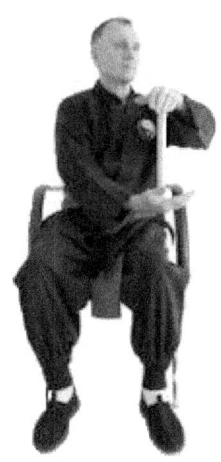

As you breathe out, *express*, as you rotate the "central core" of the body to the left, and drive your right hand under your left hand, so that the *Chi Baton*™, is vertical. (Remember to keep the hips facing forward!)

As you drive the hand under, make sure that your left hand stays where it is relative to the body, (i.e. In front of the left shoulder) so that you have to tum your central core in co-ordination with the movement.

Remember to keep your shoulders relaxed at all times.

(In this exercise, as you drive the right hand under the left, *express* with the right hand and right instep only.)

Release, as you breath in, returning to the forward facing position with the elbows spread outwards, and the *Chi Baton*™ horizontal to the floor at chest height.

Repeat the movement, reversing left and right, and then do the whole sequence another three times.

Relax the elbows and lower the arms.

Drive The Hand Over

(Although this exercise is superficially similar to the previous one, it is in fact quite different.)

In the previous exercise, the action of the body and arms compress one side of the body to expel air from the lungs.

In this exercise, the action of the body and the arms opens up the ribcage to improve the intake of air to the relevant side of the chest.

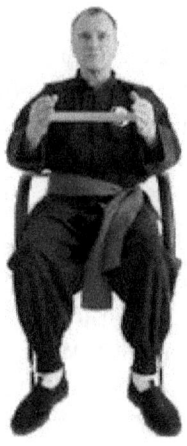

Sit comfortably, holding the baton at chest height, with the shoulders and elbows relaxed.

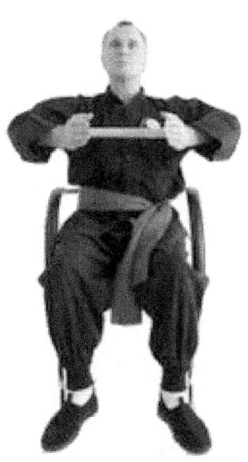

Lift both elbows gently upwards, being careful to keep the shoulders down. The forearms should almost form a straight line with the **Chi Baton™**. As you lift the elbows, draw them outwards to ensure that the shoulder blades remain spread.

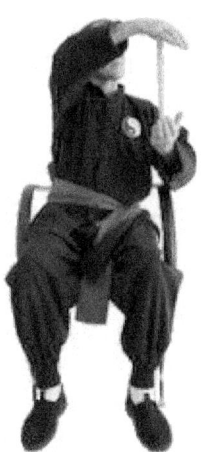

As you breathe in, **express**, as you rotate the "central core" of the body to the left, and drive your right hand **over** your left hand, so that the **Chi Baton™**, is vertical. As you drive the hand over, make sure that your left hand stays where it is relative to the body, so that you have to tum your central core to follow the movement. Remember to keep your shoulders relaxed at all times.

(In this exercise, as you drive the right hand over the left, *express* with the right hand and right instep only.)

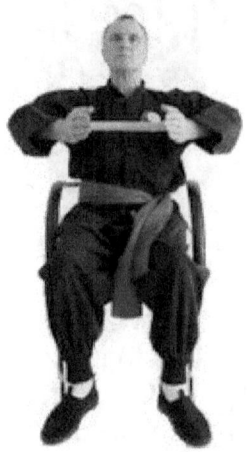

As you breath out, *release*, and return to the forward facing position with the elbows spread outwards, and the *Chi Baton*™ horizontal to the floor, at chest height.

Repeat the movement, substituting left for right.

Repeat the whole sequence another three times.

Relax the elbows and lower the arms

Disperse the Hornets

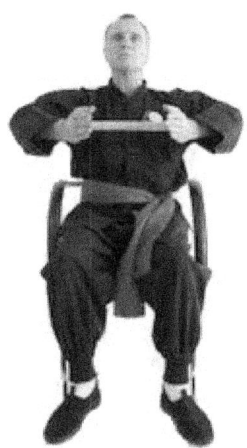

Start with the **Chi Baton™** held at the centre of your chest., about two fist distances from the body. The elbows should be raised, upwards and outwards, as if lifted by two gently inflating balloons, so that they almost form a line with the **Chi Baton™** . The shoulders should remain relaxed with shoulder blades spread.

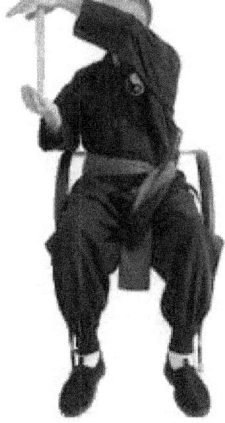

On the in breath, *express* as you lift the left arm

upwards and across the centre of the body until the left hand is vertically above the right. Remember to keep the right hand in the same position relative to the body as you make the movement, to ensure the left hand side of the ribcage has to open properly.

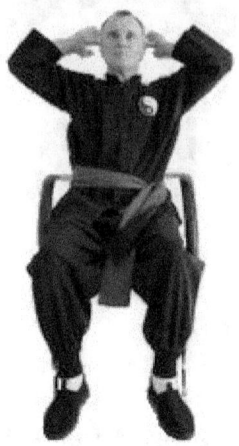

Use the right arm to drive the baton upwards and behind the head. (Be careful to keep your head upright and not to crane your chin forward). If this is too much of a stretch, finish with the **Chi Baton™** above the centre point of the head.

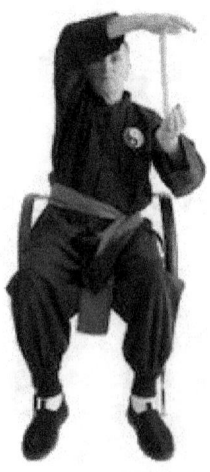

On the out breath, *release* as you lift the right arm over and across the back of the neck until the **Chi Baton™** is vertical with the right hand above the left. .

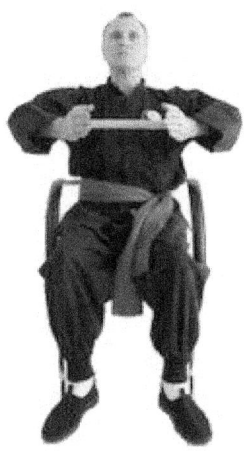

Now continue to circle the right arm forwards until you return to the start position with the **Chi Baton™** in the centre of your sternum (chest), about two fist distances from the body.

Do 6 repetitions in one direction and then reverse the instructions and do 6 repetitions in the opposite direction.

Three Section Breathing

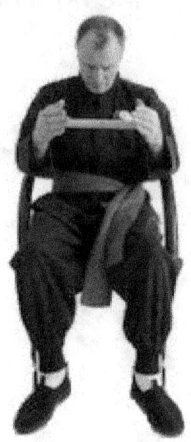

Sit holding the **Chi Baton™** in the centre of your sternum (chest), about two fist distances from the body. The elbows are relaxed and close to, but not touching, the sides of the body. The head is lifted upward, outward and downward, with the chin almost touching the chest, and the throat open and relaxed.

Breathe in, drawing air into the belly, using the diaphragm only.

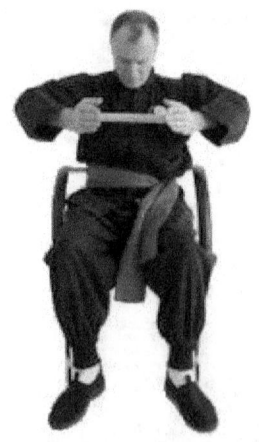

Continue to breathe in to the lower chest as you *express*, and lift both elbows gently upwards, being careful to keep the shoulders down. The forearms should almost form a straight line with the **Chi Baton**™ As you lift the elbows, draw them outwards to ensure that the shoulder blades remain spread.

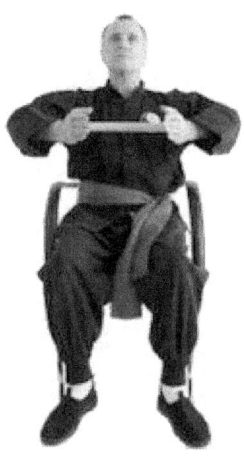

Continue to breathe in to the upper chest as you lift the sternum and raise the head to look forwards.

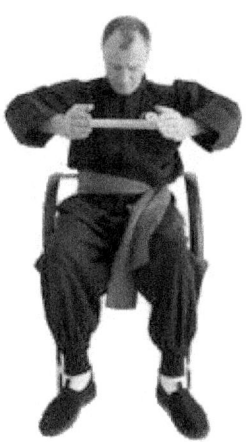

On the out breath, *release*, breathing out from the upper chest first, as you lower the head outwards and downwards.

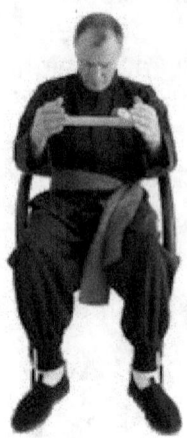

Continue to breathe out from the lower chest, as you gently lower both elbows, until they are close to, but not touching, the chest.

Continue to breath out from the belly, gently drawing the stomach in, and lifting the diaphragm upwards.

Repeat the whole sequence another three times.

Alternate Three Section Breathing

This exercise is similar to the previous one but **slightly more difficult** to perform. Be careful not to over strain when performing each section. The out breath is the same as the previous exercise.

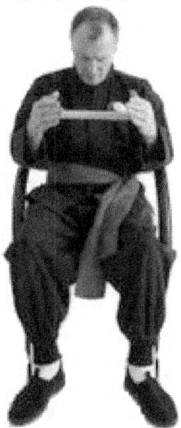

Sit holding the **Chi Baton™** in the centre of your sternum (chest), about two fist distances from the body. The elbows are relaxed and close to, but not touching, the sides of the body. The head is lifted upwards, outward and downward, with the chin almost touching the chest.

Breathe in, drawing air into the belly, using the diaphragm only.

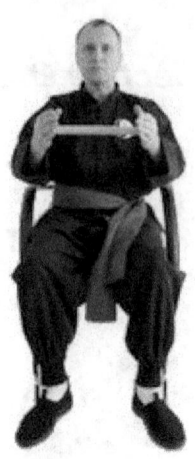

Continue to breathe in to the upper chest as you lift the sternum and raise the head to look forwards.

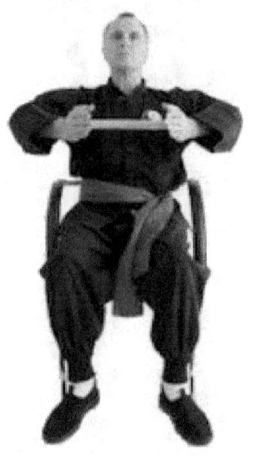

Continue to breathe in to the lower chest as you *express*, and lift both elbows gently upwards, being careful to keep the shoulders down. The forearms should almost form a straight line with the **Chi Baton™**. As you lift the elbows, draw them outwards to ensure that the shoulder blades remain spread.

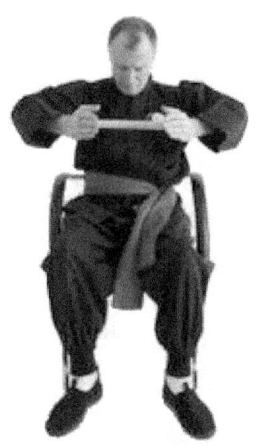

On the out breath, *release*, breathing out from the upper chest first, as you lower the head outwards and downwards.

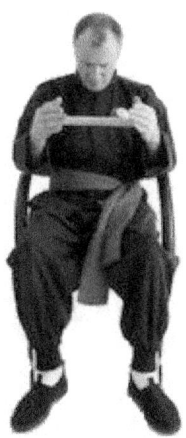

Continue to breathe out from the lower chest, as you gently lower both elbows, until they are close to, but not touching, the chest.

Continue to breath out from the belly, gently drawing the stomach in, and lifting the diaphragm upwards.

Repeat the whole sequence another three times.

Double Expectations

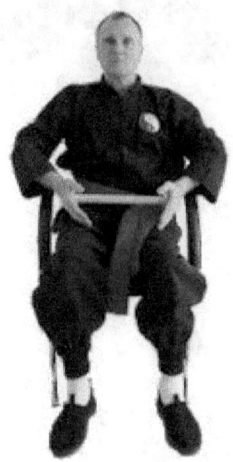

Sit comfortably, with arms relaxed.

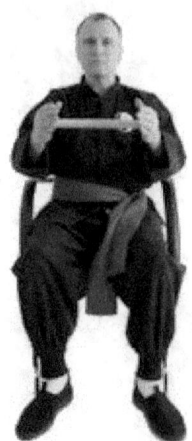

On the in breath, *express,* as you circle the **Chi Baton**™ forwards and upwards. As the elbows pass in front of the body, draw them in, as if holding a second **Chi Baton**™ between them.

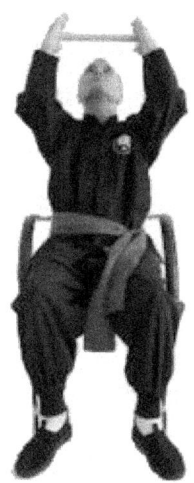

Keep the elbows in this shape for the rest of the in breath, until it finishes above the head.

Remember not to raise the shoulders as you do so, but generate the movement by rolling the shoulder joint in its socket.

As the baton passes in front of the eyes, follow its progress, allowing the chin to draw forward slightly to prevent the blood vessels from being restricted, and the back of the neck from being compressed.

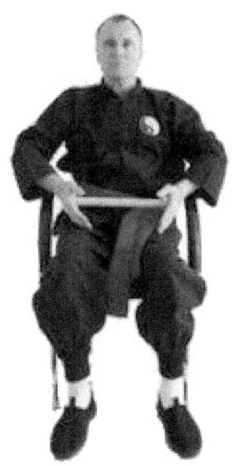

On the out breath, *release*, and return to the start position. The out breath should be longer than the in breath. (If the in breath takes four seconds then the out breath should take six.)

Repeat the whole sequence another three times.

Double Expectations With Spread Elbows

Sit comfortably, with arms relaxed.

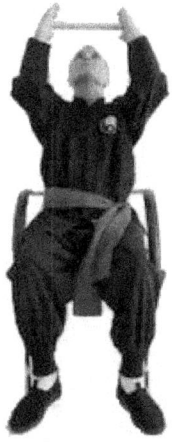

On the in breath, *express*, and circle the **Chi Baton**™ forwards and upwards until it finishes above the head. Remember not to raise the shoulders as you do so, but generate the movement by rolling the shoulder joint in its socket.

As the elbows pass in front of the body, draw them in, as if holding a further **Chi Baton**™ between them.

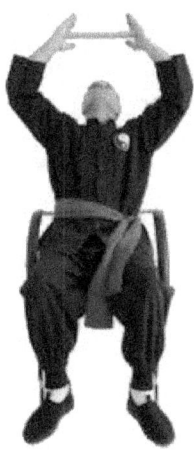

Hold the elbows in this position until you have reached your maximum position and then spread the elbows sideways for the rest of the in breath, (Be careful to draw the elbows sideways and not back, as taking the elbows back will close the shoulder blades and cut off the flow of energy.).

As before, when the baton passes in front of the eyes, follow its progress, allowing the chin to draw forward slightly to prevent the blood vessels from being restricted.

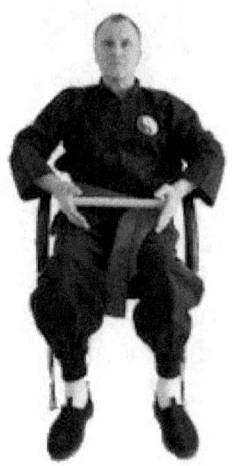

On the out breath, *release*, and allow the elbows to relax inwards, before returning to the start position. The out breath should be longer than the in breath. (If the in breath takes four seconds then the out breath should take six.)

Repeat the whole sequence another three times.

Advanced Double Expectations.

(Important! Do not attempt the advanced version of Double Expectations, until you have practised the previous versions for at least six months, regularly!!)

The movements in this exercise are the same as the simple version of double expectations with the differences *in italics*.

On the in breath, **express**, and **snort in four strong, sharp in breaths, through the nose,** as you drive the **Chi Baton**™ forwards and upwards, with each sniff, until it finishes above the head. Remember not to raise the shoulders as you do so, but generate the movement by rolling the shoulder joint in its socket.

As before, when the elbows pass in front of the body, draw them in, as if holding a further **Chi Baton**™ between them. Keep the elbows in this shape for the rest of the in breath.

As the baton passes in front of the eyes, follow its progress, allowing the chin to draw forward slightly to prevent the blood vessels from being restricted.

On the out breath, **release,** and allow the elbows to return to the start position. The out breath should be continuous, and longer than the in breath. (If the in breath takes four seconds then the out breath should take six.)

Repeat the whole sequence another three times.

Raise One Side

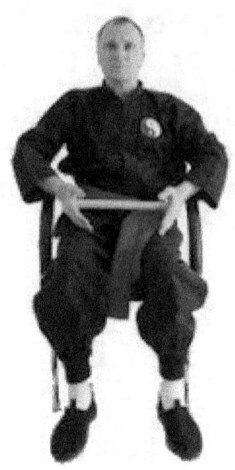

Sit comfortably, with the spine straight and feet flat on the floor.

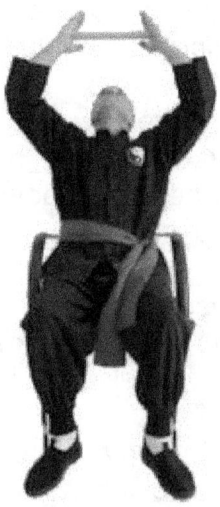

On the in breath, gently raise the arms outwards and upwards, spreading the shoulder blades and elbows as you do so, until they are above the head. Remember not to raise the shoulders, but generate the movement by rolling the shoulder joint in its socket. As usual, follow the upward path of the baton with your eyes.

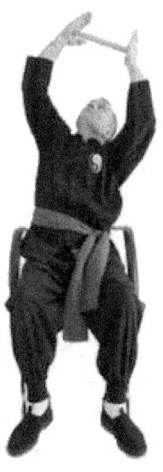

On the out breath, *express*, and extend the right hand side of the body, so the right hand lifts slightly above the left. The movement is performed wholly with the area between the shoulder and the hip. Be careful not to raise the shoulders, straighten the right arm, or compress the opposite side of the body.

(In this exercise, as you extend the right hand side of the body, *express* with the right hand and right instep only.)

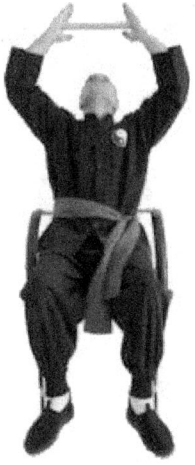

On the in breath, *release*, and straighten the spine.

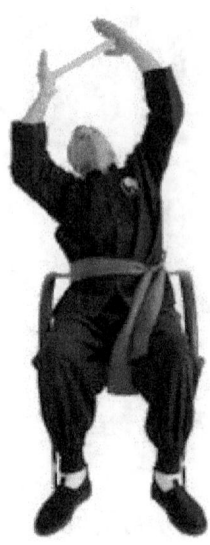

On the out breath, ***express***, and extend the left hand side of the body, so the left hand lifts above the right.

(As you extend the left hand side of the body, ***express*** with the left hand and left instep only.)

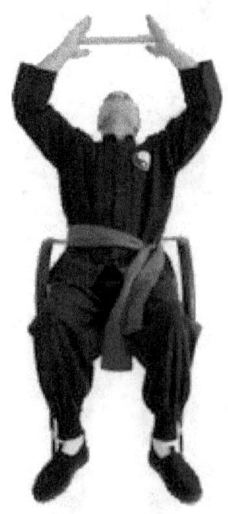

On the in breath, ***release***, and straighten the spine.

On the out breath, gently lower the arms to the start position.

Repeat the whole sequence another three times.

Spinal Twists

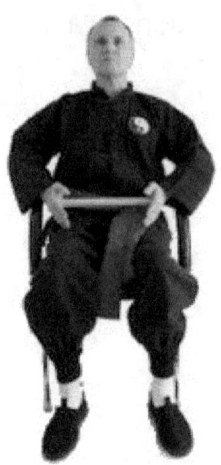

Sit comfortably, with the spine straight and feet flat on the floor.

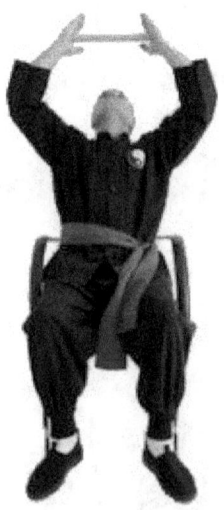

On the in breath, gently raise the arms outwards and upwards, spreading the shoulder blades and elbows as you do so, until the are above the head. Remember not to raise the shoulders, but generate the movement by rolling the shoulder joint in its socket. As usual, follow the upward path of the baton with your eyes.

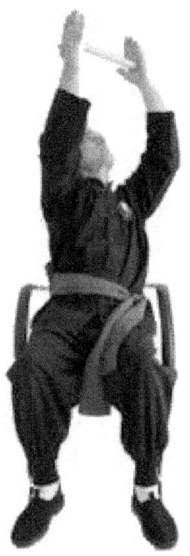

On the out breath, **express**, and extend the spine, twisting the "central core" of the body to the left as you do so. Be careful not to raise the shoulders or straighten the arms. Relax the elbows so that they point forwards as you do so.

(In this exercise, as you twist to the left, **express,** with both hands and right instep only.)

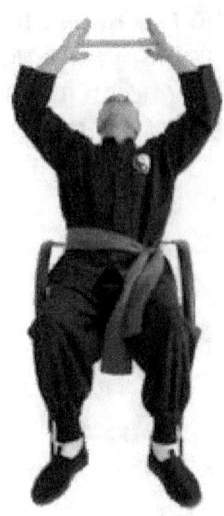

On the in breath, *release*, and turn the body to the front. Spread the shoulders and elbows as you do so.

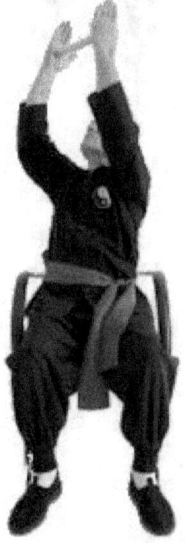

On the out breath, *express*, and extend the spine, twisting the central core of the body to the right as you do so. Be careful not to raise the shoulders or straighten the arms. Relax the elbows so that they point forwards as you do so.

(As you twist to the right, **express,** with both hands and left instep only.)

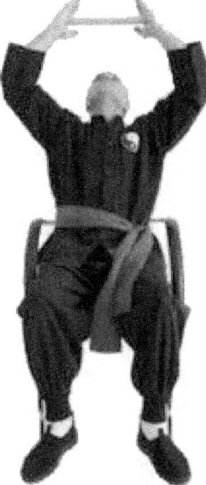

On the in breath, **release**, and turn the body to the front. Spread the shoulders and elbows as you do so.

On the out breath, gently lower the arms to the start position.

Repeat the whole sequence another three times.

Spinal Twists With Lean.

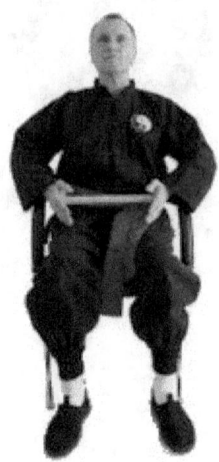

Sit comfortably, with the spine straight and feet flat on the floor.

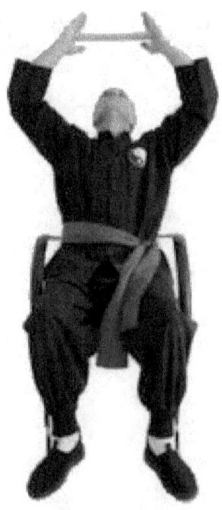

On the in breath, gently raise the arms outwards and upwards, spreading the shoulder blades and elbows as you do so, until the are above the head. Remember not to raise the shoulders, but generate the movement by rolling the shoulder joint in its socket.

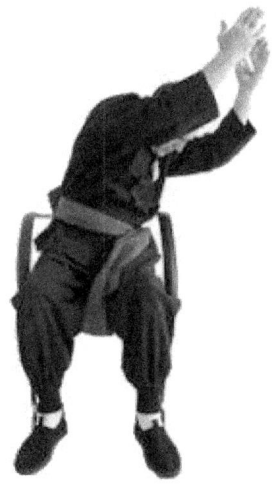

On the out breath, **express**, and extend the spine, twisting the "central core" of the body to the left as you do so. Be careful not to raise the shoulders or straighten the arms.

At the same time, lean to the left, by bending from the hips. Be careful not to over strain, and keep the head in the same position relative to the arms. Relax the elbows so that they point forwards and slightly downwards as you do so.

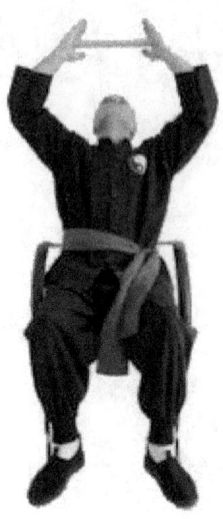

On the in breath, ***release***, and straighten the spine. Spread the elbows and shoulders as you do so.

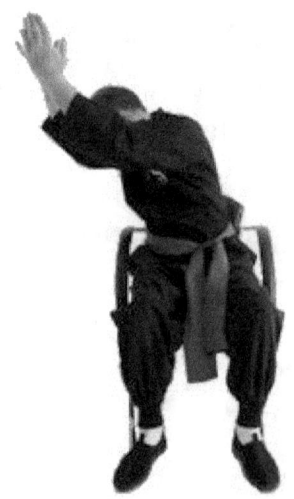

On the out breath, ***express***, and extend the spine, twisting the "central" core of the body to the right as you do so. Be careful not to raise the shoulders or straighten the arms.

At the same time, lean to the right, being careful not to over strain and keeping the head in the same position relative to the arms. Relax the elbows so that they point forwards and slightly down as you do so.

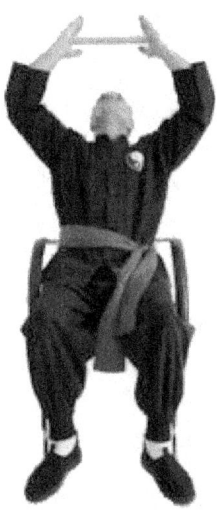

On the in breath, *release*, and straighten the spine, spreading the elbows and shoulders.

On the out breath, gently lower the arms to the start position.

Repeat the whole sequence another three times.

Push Mountains

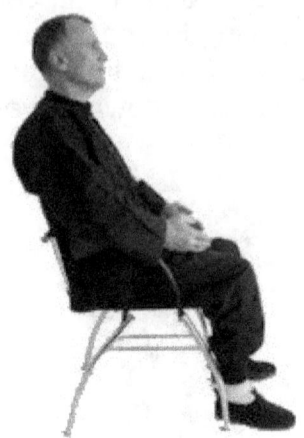

Sit comfortably, with the body erect and feet flat on the floor.

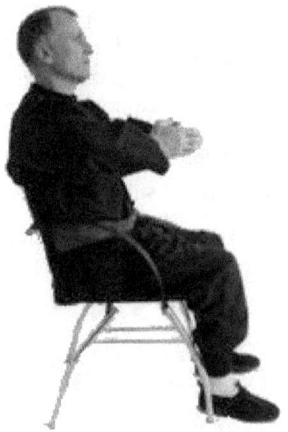

On the in breath, gently raise the **Chi Baton™** until it lines up two fist distances from the centre of the chest. Spread the shoulder blades and elbows outwards as you do so. Remember not to raise the shoulders.

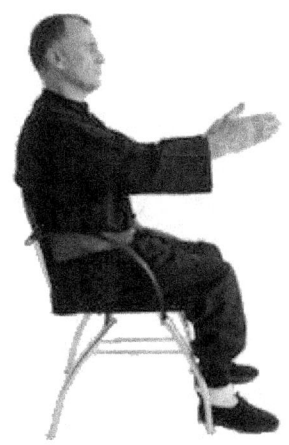

On the out breath, *express*, and extend the arms forwards, allowing the elbows to drop until they are pointing downwards. Be careful to keep the shoulders in their sockets and not to allow them to drift forwards.

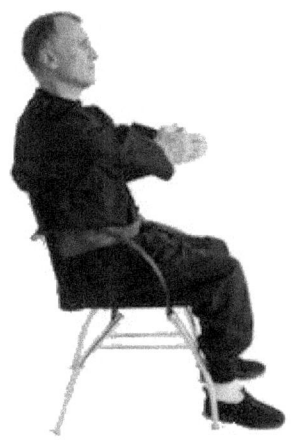

On the in breath, *release,* and gently extend the elbows outwards to draw the **Chi Baton™** inwards again, until it lines up with the centre of the chest.

(Remember to keep the **Chi Baton™** two fist distances from the chest).

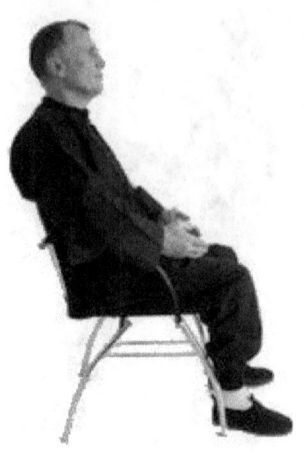

On the out breath, gently lower the arms.

Repeat the whole sequence another three times.

Push Mountains and Lean Forward

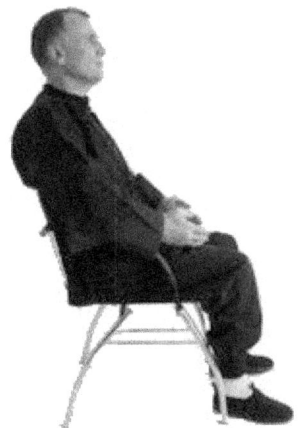

Sit comfortably, with the spine straight and feet flat on the floor.

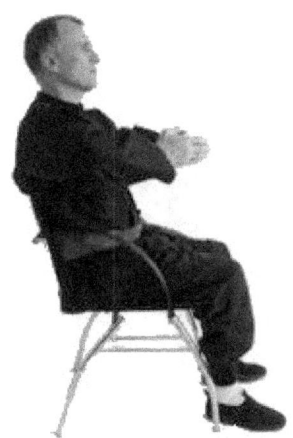

On the in breath, gently raise the **Chi Baton™** until it lines up two fist distances from the centre of the chest. Spread the shoulder blades and elbows outwards as you do so. Remember not to raise the shoulders.

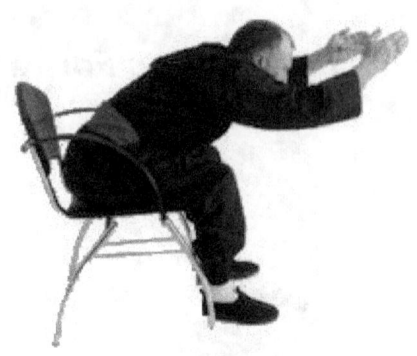

On the out breath, **express**, and extend the arms forwards, allowing the elbows to drop until they are pointing downwards. Be careful to keep the shoulders in their sockets and not to allow them to drift forwards, and keep the head in line with the body. At the same time, extend the spine, and lower the body so that it finishes horizontal to the floor, in between the arms. (The chin drifts forwards slightly to relieve the pressure on the blood vessels of the neck).

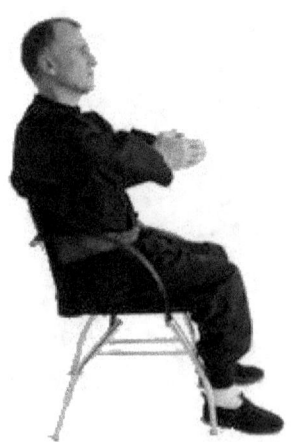

On the in breath, **release,** raise the body upright again, and gently extend the elbows outwards to draw the **Chi Baton™** inwards again, until it lines up with the centre of the chest.

(Remember to keep the **Chi Baton™** two fist

distances from the chest).

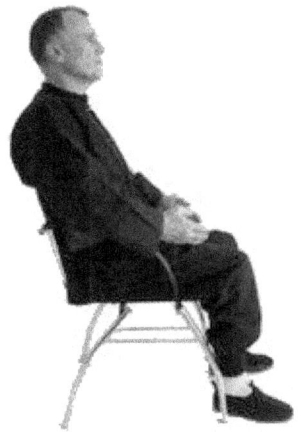

On the out breath, gently lower the arms.

Repeat the whole sequence another three times.

Heel Lifts

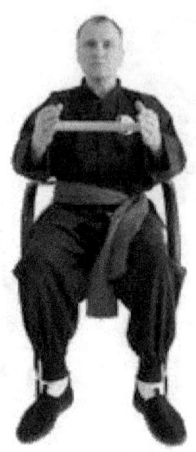

Sit comfortably, with the spine straight and feet flat on the floor. With the **Chi Baton™** lined up with, and two fist distances from, the centre of the chest. The shoulders are relaxed with the elbows pointing downwards.

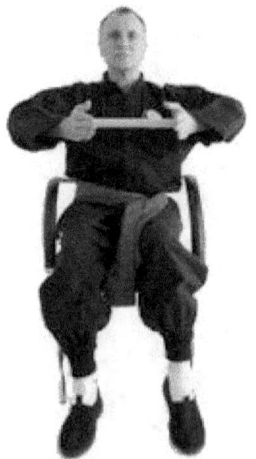

On the in breath, **express**, with hands and right foot, as you spread the shoulder blades and elbows outwards. At the same time raise the left heel as high as you comfortably can.

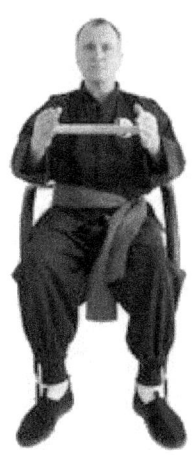

On the in breath, *release*, and return to the front facing position, with the elbows relaxed, pointing down, and the centre of the **Chi Baton™** lined up with the centre of the chest.

Repeat the movement on the opposite side.

Do the whole sequence, both sides, another three times.

Toe Lifts

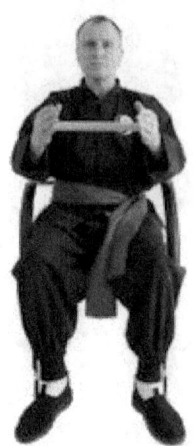

Sit comfortably, with the **Chi Baton™** two fist distances from the centre of the chest. The shoulders are relaxed with the elbows pointing downwards.

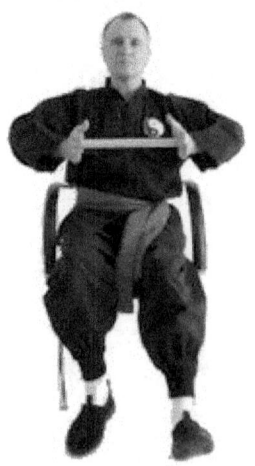

On the in breath, *express* with both hands and right foot as you spread the shoulder blades and elbows outwards. At the same time, strongly slide the left heel forwards, allowing the toes to lift, so that they point upwards.

(N.B. Do not just pull the toes upwards, as this will cramp the front of the leg and close the front of the ankle joint! Allow the toes to rise by the forward action of the heel.)

On the in breath, *release*, and return to the previous position, by relaxing the foot and allowing the foot to draw back. The elbows relax, pointing down, and the centre of the **Chi Baton**™ lines up with the centre of the chest.

Repeat the movement to the right hand side.

Do the whole sequence, both sides, another three times.

Knee Lifts

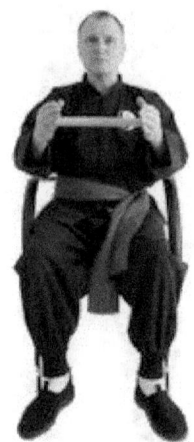

Sit comfortably. The **Chi Baton™** is lined up with, and two fist distances from, the centre of the chest. The elbows are relaxed and point downwards.

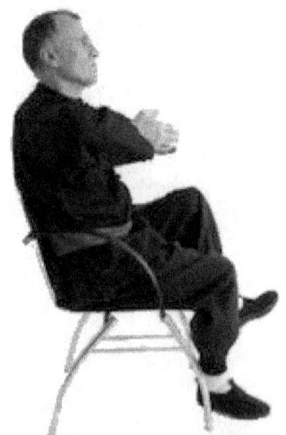

On the in breath, *express*, and spread the shoulder blades and elbows outwards. At the same time lift the left knee upwards, keeping the foot flat, parallel to the ground,. (i.e. Not pointing the toe!)

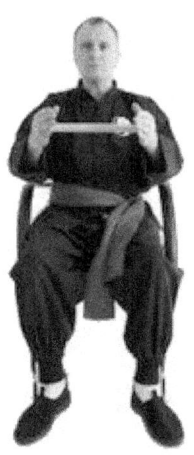

On the out breath, *release,* and return to the start position.

N.B. As you raise the knee, and *express,* remember to slightly raise the arch of the supporting foot. (i.e. The foot resting on the floor).

Repeat the above, substituting right for left etc.

Do the whole sequence, both sides, another three times.

Leg Straightening

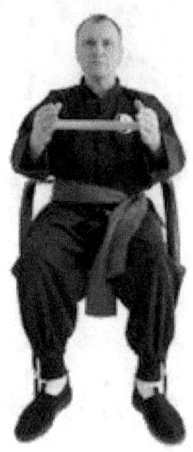

Sit comfortably, with the **Chi Baton™** lined up with, and two fist distances from, the centre of the chest. The elbows are relaxed and point downwards.

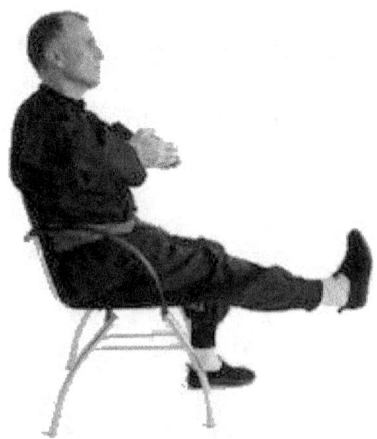

On the in breath, *express*, with both hands and supporting foot, and spread the shoulder blades and elbows outwards. At the same time straighten the left leg upwards, without locking the knee, and expressing through the heel of the foot so that you finish with the leg straight and toe pointing to the ceiling.

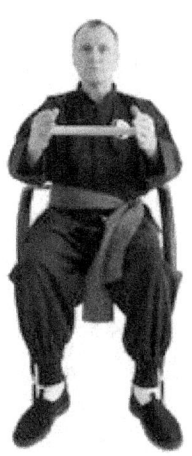

On the out breath, *release,* and return to the start position.

Repeat the above, this time with the right leg.
Do the whole sequence, both sides, another three times.

Knee Lifts and Straightens

(This is a mixture of the previous two exercises.)

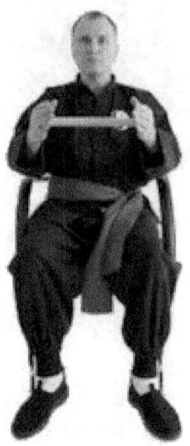

Sit comfortably, with the spine straight and feet flat on the floor. With the **Chi Baton™** lined up with the centre of the chest. The elbows are relaxed and point downwards.

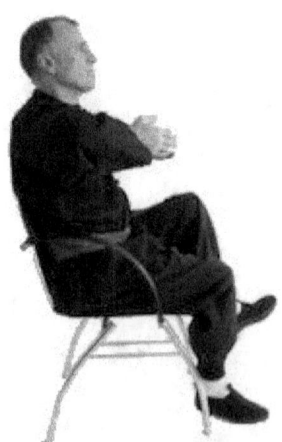

On the in breath, spread the shoulder blades and elbows outwards. At the same time lift the left knee.

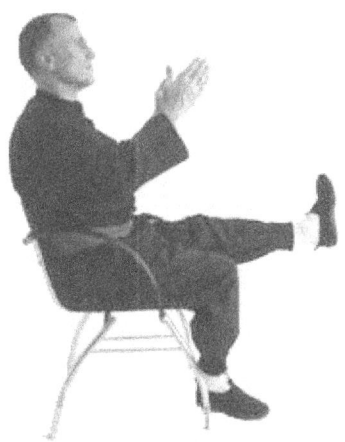

On the out breath, **express**, as you straighten the left leg, without locking the knee, and extending through the heel of the foot so that you finish with the leg straight and toe pointing to the ceiling.

At the same time relax the elbows so that they point downwards and slightly lengthen the arms, but without allowing the shoulders to move forward in the shoulder socket.

N.B. As you raise the leg, and **express,** remember to slightly raise the instep of the supporting foot. (i.e. The foot resting on the floor).

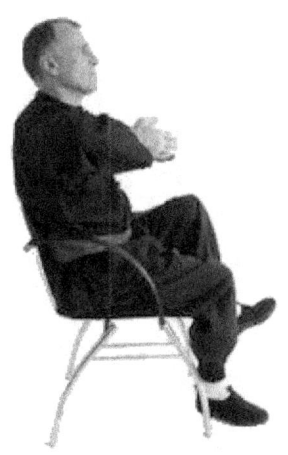

As you breathe in, **Release,** and bend the knee, spreading the shoulders as you do so.

Lower the leg and return to the start position.

Repeat the above, with the right leg.

Repeat the whole sequence, both sides, another three times.

Hip Opens

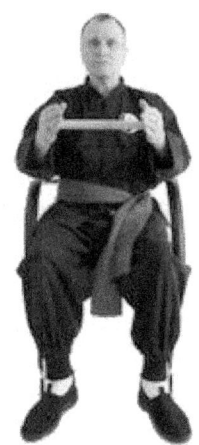

Sit comfortably, with the **Chi Baton**™ lined up with, and two fist distances from, the centre of the chest. The shoulders are relaxed with the elbows pointing downwards.

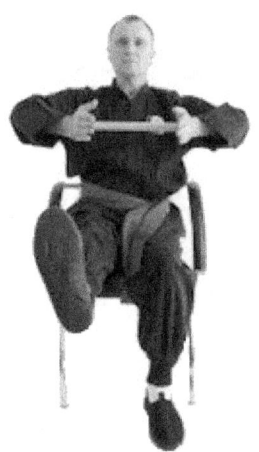

On the in breath, spread the shoulder blades and elbows outwards. At the same time lift the left leg, extending through the heel, without locking the knee.

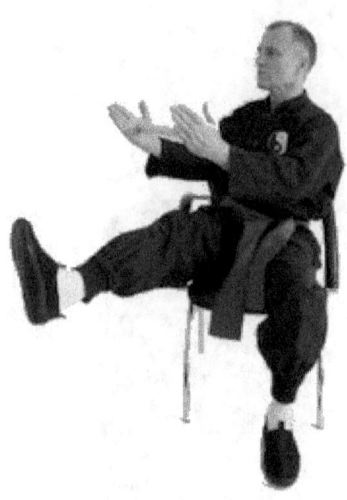

On the out breath, **express**, with both hands and supporting leg, as you rotate the "central core" of the body to the right, and open the left hip so that the leg and body move to the right. Relax the elbows so that they point down as you do so. (The pressure remains the same on both buttocks.)

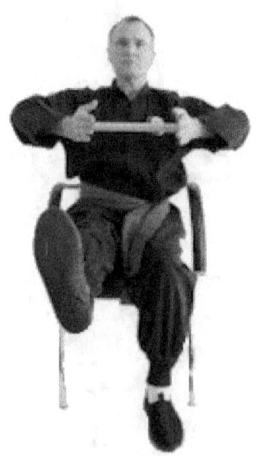

On the in breath, **release**, and return to the front facing position, with the elbows spread.

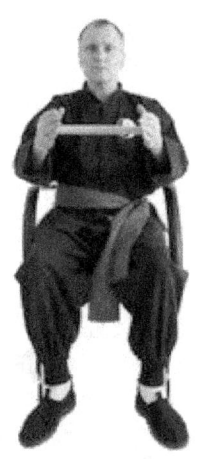

On the next out breath, lower the arms and leg simultaneously.

Repeat the above, with the right leg.

Do the whole sequence, both sides, another three times.

Waist Turns With Arm Extensions

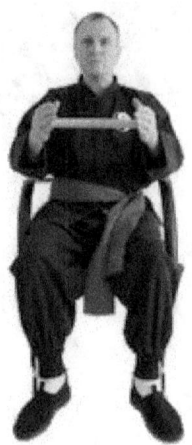

Sit comfortably. The **Chi Baton™** is lined up with, and two fist distances from, the centre of the chest. The shoulders are relaxed with the elbows pointing downwards.

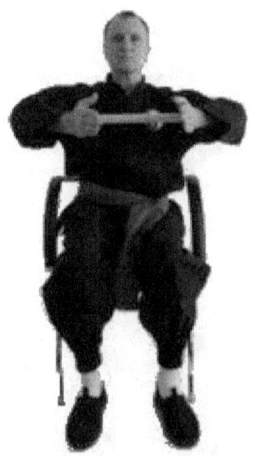

On the in breath, spread the shoulder blades and elbows outwards.

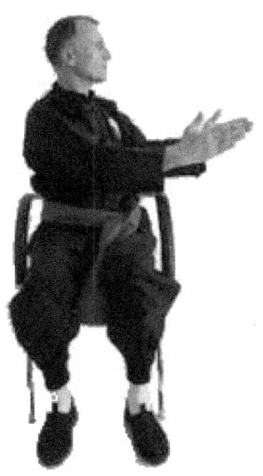

On the out breath, **express**, as you lift and rotate the "central core" of the body to the left. Relax the elbows so that they point down as you do so, and extend the hands forward a little way by slightly straightening the elbows. Be careful not to move the shoulder joint forward in its socket as you do so.

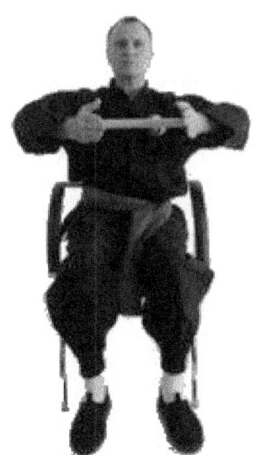

On the in breath, **release**, and return to the front facing position, with the elbows spread.

Repeat the movement to the right hand side.

On the in breath, *release*, and return to the front facing position, with the elbows spread.

On the out breath, relax the elbows so that they point down.

Do the whole sequence, both sides, another three times.

Growing Pine

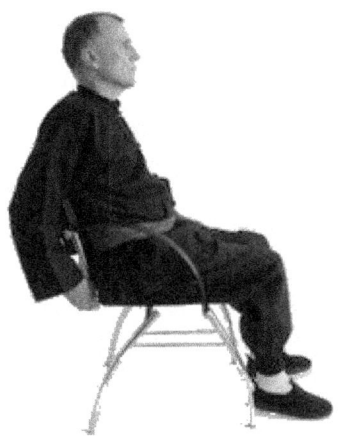

Sit comfortably, with the spine straight and feet flat on the floor. Hold the **Chi Baton**™ behind the chair with the fingers pointing down

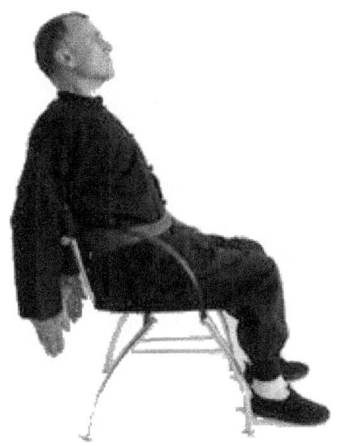

On the in breath, ***express***, as you extend your arms downwards and outwards. At the same time, lift the centre of the chest (sternum), upwards, and lengthen the whole spine as if you were trying to touch the

ceiling with the crown of your head. (N.B. As you do this you should feel your chin draw in slightly, as if performing a very small nodding action. Also, remember, as with any of the **Chi Baton**™ exercises, attempt to keep the shoulders open, and do not allow the shoulder blades to draw together or touch!)

On the out breath, *release,* and return to the start position.

Repeat the whole sequence, another three times

Sit Still

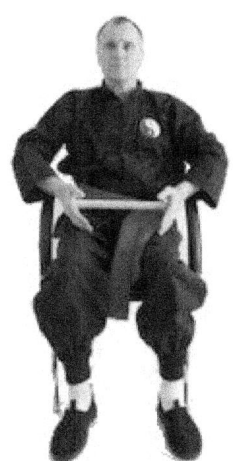

Sit comfortably, holding the *Chi Baton*™ at belly height, one fist distance from the body, with the shoulders relaxed and elbows gently extended sideways. Keep the tongue on the roof of the mouth and focus on circulating energy from the belly down the left arm, across the *Chi Baton*™, up the right arm and back to the belly, making a clockwise circle.

Do this for at least one minute, circulating the energy clockwise, and then repeat the exercise for at least one minute, circulating the energy anti-clockwise.

Close the Fountain

(This exercise is the reverse of **Open the Fountain**, at the start of the programme.)

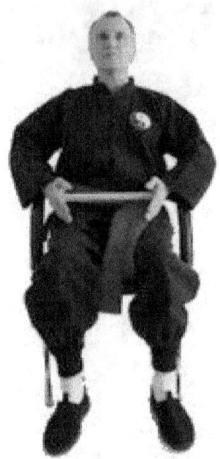

Sit comfortably, with the shoulders and elbows relaxed.

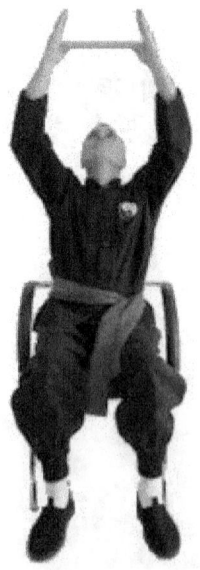

As you breathe in, **express** , as you roll the shoulders, to lift the **Chi Baton**™ gently forwards and upwards, away from the body, in a curving motion, until it is above, and slightly to the front of, the head.

As you lift the **Chi Baton**™ gently upwards, draw the elbows outwards, allowing the shoulder blades to spread, so that the back is fully open. Follow the movement of the **Chi Baton**™ with your eyes as it travels past and above your face. Allow the chin to drift forwards a little as you do so to ensure the blood vessels in the neck are kept free and open.

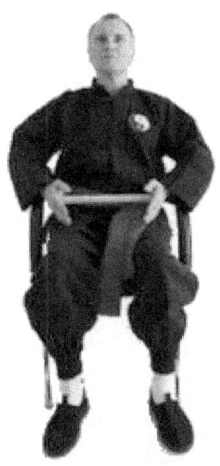

As you breathe out, **release**, in a controlled manner, and return to the start position, by allowing the elbows to relax inwards, and then drawing the hands directly down in front of, and one fist distance away from, the body.

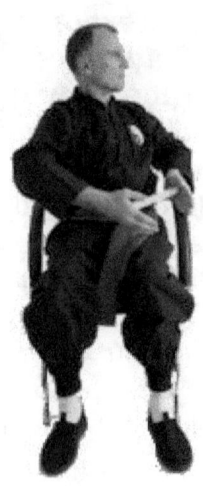

Turn the central core of your body, gently, to the left.

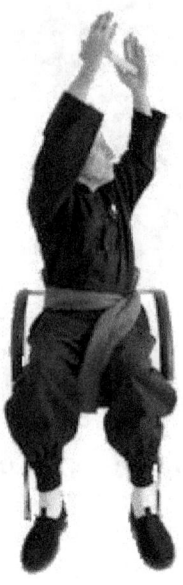

Keeping the body turned, breathe in and, *express*, as before, as you lift the *Chi Baton*™ gently upwards, in a curving arc, until it is above and slightly to the front of the head.

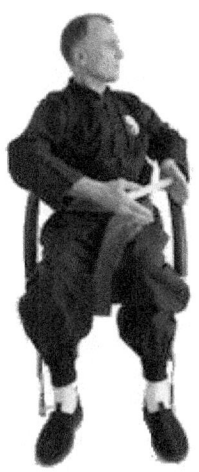

As you breathe out, *release*, in the controlled manner outlined previously, and return to the start position,

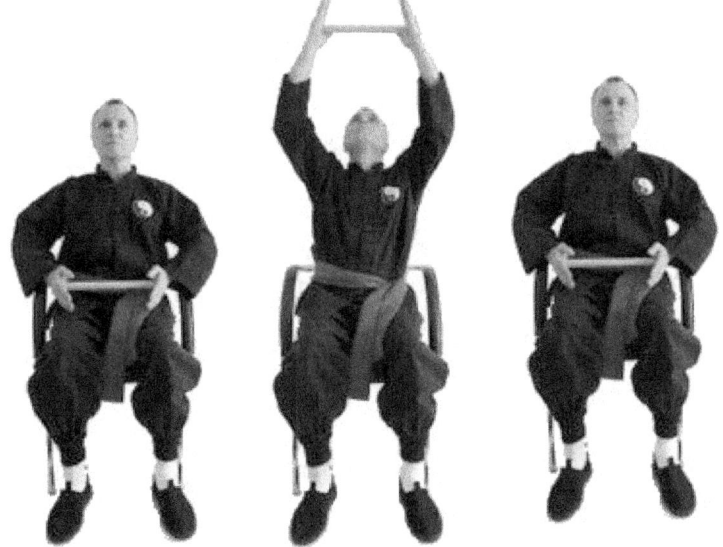

Turn back to the front position, and perform another repetition of the movement to the front.

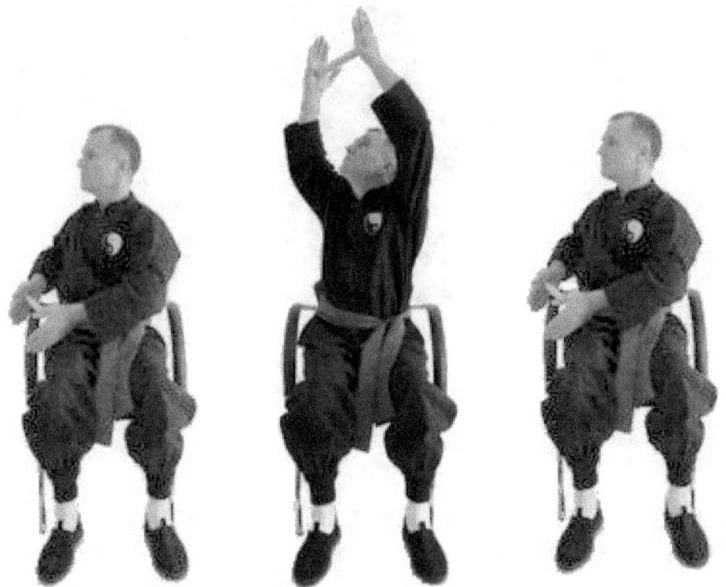

Turn the central core of your body, gently, to the right and perform another repetition of the movement to the right hand side.

Turn back to the front position, and perform another repetition of the movement to the front.

Repeat the whole sequence outlined above three times more.

Relax and enjoy the glow of energy as it travels around the body.

If you enjoyed this book, you may like to know of other **Chi Baton**™ publications, by **Barry Westley.**.

For more information, or if you have any questions you would like clarified, contact the web site:

www.chibaton.co.uk

TM ©

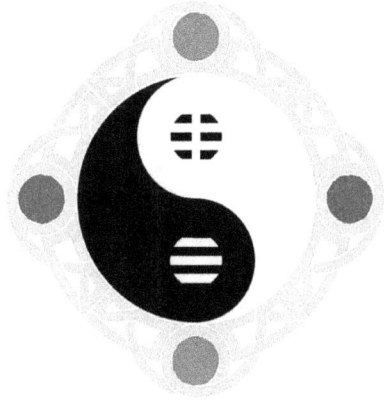

Barry Westley 2014 ©

www.ingramcontent.com/pod-product-compliance
Lightning Source LLC
Chambersburg PA
CBHW071354310526
45790CB00017B/627

* 9 7 8 1 5 0 2 7 1 8 6 0 0 *